GW01158539

The Ultimate Mediterranean Diet Recipe Collection for Beginners

Fast and Affordable Recipes to Burn Your Fats and Start Eating Healthy

Lexi Robertson

© **Copyright 2021 - All rights reserved.**

The content contained within this book may not be reproduced, duplicated or transmitted without direct written permission from the author or the publisher.

Under no circumstances will any blame or legal responsibility be held against the publisher, or author, for any damages, reparation, or monetary loss due to the information contained within this book. Either directly or indirectly.

Legal Notice:

This book is copyright protected. This book is only for personal use. You cannot amend, distribute, sell, use, quote or paraphrase any part, or the content within this book, without the consent of the author or publisher.

Disclaimer Notice:

Please note the information contained within this document is for educational and entertainment purposes only. All effort has been executed to present accurate, up to date, and reliable, complete information. No warranties of any kind are declared or implied. Readers acknowledge that the author is not engaging in the rendering of legal, financial, medical or professional advice. The content within this book has been derived from various sources. Please consult a licensed professional before attempting any techniques outlined in this book.

By reading this document, the reader agrees that under no circumstances is the author responsible for any losses, direct or indirect, which are incurred as a result of the use of information contained within this document, including, but not limited to, — errors, omissions, or inaccuracies.

Table of contents

BROILED TOMATOES WITH FETA 7

MEDITERRANEAN LAMB CHOPS 10

BROILED MUSHROOMS BURGERS AND GOAT CHEESE 12

TUNA AND POTATO SALAD 14

WILD RICE SOUP & CREAMY CHICKEN 16

GARLIC RICE 18

CARROT RICE 20

PASTA SALAD WITH CHICKEN CLUB 21

TOMATO CREAM SAUCE 23

ALFREDO PEPPERED SHRIMP 25

PESTO WITH BASIL AND SPINACH 28

BLACKENED SALMON FILLETS 30

TASTY CRABBY PANINI 34

BEAN AND TOASTED PITA SALAD 37

GOAT CHEESE 'N RED BEANS SALAD 39

SPICY SWEET RED HUMMUS 41

DILL RELISH ON WHITE SEA BASS 42

VEGETABLE LOVER'S CHICKEN SOUP 44

MUSTARD CHOPS WITH APRICOT-BASIL RELISH 46

SEAFOOD AND VEGGIE PASTA 48

CREAMY ALFREDO FETTUCCINE 51

TASTY LASAGNA ROLLS 52

TORTELLINI SALAD WITH BROCCOLI 54

SIMPLE PENNE ANTI-PASTO 56

BUTTERNUT SQUASH HUMMUS 59

PARMESAN MASHED POTATOES WITH OLIVE OIL, GARLIC, & PARSLEY 62

- GREEK CAULIFLOWER RICE WITH FETA AND OLIVES 64
- BRUSSELS SPROUTS 66
- GARLIC SCAPES SAUTÉED WITH OLIVE OIL, SEA SALT & FRESHLY GROUND PEPPER 68
- JULENE'S GREEN JUICE 70
- CHOCOLATE BANANA SMOOTHIE 73
- FRUIT SMOOTHIE 74
- CHIA-POMEGRANATE SMOOTHIE 76
- SWEET KALE SMOOTHIE 77
- AVOCADO-BLUEBERRY SMOOTHIE 79
- CRANBERRY-PUMPKIN SMOOTHIE 80
- SWEET CRANBERRY NECTAR 81
- HEARTY PEAR AND MANGO SMOOTHIE 82
- FIG SMOOTHIE WITH CINNAMON 83
- BREAKFAST ALMOND MILK SHAKE 84
- RASPBERRY VANILLA SMOOTHIE 85
- BLUEBERRY BANANA PROTEIN SMOOTHIE 86
- HONEY AND WILD BLUEBERRY SMOOTHIE 87
- OATS BERRY SMOOTHIE 88
- KALE-PINEAPPLE SMOOTHIE 89
- MOROCCAN AVOCADO SMOOTHIE 90
- MEDITERRANEAN SMOOTHIE 91
- ANTI-INFLAMMATORY BLUEBERRY SMOOTHIE 92
- PINA COLADA SMOOTHIE 93
- KIWI SMOOTHIE 94
- WHOLE BAKED WITH LEMON AND HERBS 96
- SKILLET COD WITH FRESH TOMATO SALSA 98
- BROILED FLOUNDER WITH NECTARINE AND WHITE BEAN SALSA 100

TROUT WITH RUBY RED GRAPEFRUIT RELISH 102

CLASSIC PORK TENDERLOIN MARSALA 104

CHILI-SPICED LAMB CHOPS 106

GREEK HERBED BEEF MEATBALLS 108

SAUTÉED DARK LEAFY GREENS 111

Broiled Tomatoes with Feta

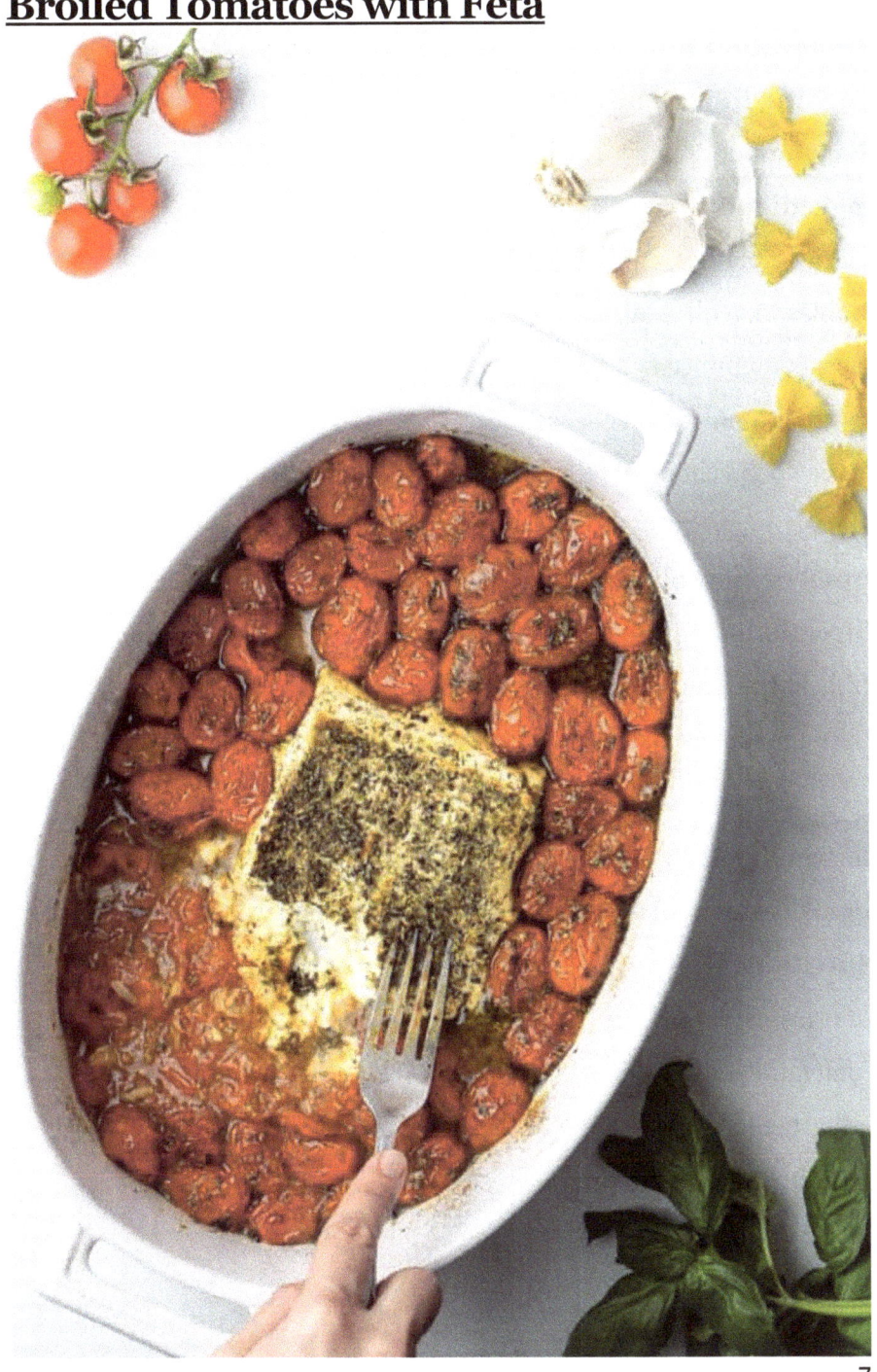

Difficulty Level: 2/5

Preparation time: 10 minutes

Cooking time: 8 minutes

Servings: 4

Ingredients:

4 large tomatoes, cut in half horizontally

1 tablespoon olive oil

1 teaspoon minced garlic

½ cup crumbled feta cheese

1 tablespoon chopped fresh basil

Sea salt

Freshly ground black pepper

Directions:

Preheat the oven to broil.

Place the tomato halves, cut-side up, in a 9-by-13-inch baking dish and drizzle them with the olive oil. Rub the garlic into the tomatoes.

Broil the tomatoes for about 5 minutes, until softened. Sprinkle with the feta cheese and broil for 3 minutes longer.

Sprinkle with basil and season with salt and pepper. Serve.

Nutrition:

Calories: 113

Total fat: 8g

Saturated fat: 3g

Carbohydrates: 8g

Sugar: 6g

Fiber: 2g

Protein: 4g

Mediterranean Lamb Chops

Difficulty Level: 2/5

Preparation time: 10 minutes

Cooking time: 10 minute

Servings: 4

Ingredients

4 lamb shoulder chops, 8 ounce each

2 tablespoons Dijon mustard

2 tablespoons Balsamic vinegar

1 tablespoon garlic, chopped

½ cup olive oil

2 tablespoons shredded fresh basil

Directions:

Pat your lamb chop dry using kitchen towel and arrange them on a shallow glass baking dish.

Take a bowl and whisk in Dijon mustard, balsamic vinegar, garlic, pepper and mix well.

Whisk in the oil very slowly into the marinade until the mixture is smooth.

Stir in basil.

Pour the marinade over the lamb chops and stir to coat both sides well.

Cover the chops and allow them to marinate for 1-4 hours (chilled).

Take the chops out and leave them for 30 minutes to allow the temperature to reach normal level.

Pre-heat your grill to medium heat and add oil to the grate.

Grill the lamb chops for 5-10 minutes per side until both sides are browned.

Once the center of the chop reads 145 degree Fahrenheit, the chops are ready, serve and enjoy!

Nutrition (Per Serving)

Calories: 521

Fat: 45g

Carbohydrates: 3.5g

Protein: 22g

Broiled Mushrooms Burgers and Goat Cheese

Difficulty Level: 2/5

Preparation time: 15 minutes

Cooking time: 5 minutes

Servings: 4

Ingredients:

4 large Portobello mushroom caps

1 red onion, cut into ¼ inch thick slices

2 tablespoons extra virgin olive oil

2 tablespoons balsamic vinegar

Pinch of salt

¼ cup goat cheese

¼ cup sun-dried tomatoes, chopped

4 ciabatta buns

1 cup kale, shredded

Directions:

Pre-heat your oven to broil.

Take a large bowl and add mushrooms caps, onion slices, olive oil, balsamic vinegar and salt.

Mix well.

Place mushroom caps (bottom side up) and onion slices on your baking sheet.

Take a small bowl and stir in goat cheese and sun dried tomatoes.

Toast the buns under the broiler for 30 seconds until golden.

Spread the goat cheese mix on top of each bun.

Place mushroom cap and onion slice on each bun bottom and cover with shredded kale.

Put everything together and serve.

Enjoy!

Nutrition (Per Serving)

Calories: 327

Fat: 11g

Carbohydrates: 49g

Protein: 11g

Tuna and Potato Salad

Difficulty Level: 2/5

Preparation time: 10 minutes

Cooking time: nil

Servings: 4

Ingredients

1 pound baby potatoes, scrubbed, boiled

1 cup tuna chunks, drained

1 cup cherry tomatoes, halved

1 cup medium onion, thinly sliced

8 pitted black olives

2 medium hard-boiled eggs, sliced

1 head Romaine lettuce

Honey lemon mustard dressing

¼ cup olive oil

2 tablespoons lemon juice

1 tablespoon Dijon mustard

1 teaspoon dill weed, chopped

Salt as needed

Pepper as needed

Directions:

Take a small glass bowl and mix in your olive oil, honey, lemon juice, Dijon mustard and dill.

Season the mix with pepper and salt.

Add in the tuna, baby potatoes, cherry tomatoes, red onion, green beans, black olives and toss. everything nicely.

Arrange your lettuce leaves on a beautiful serving dish to make the base of your salad.

Top them with your salad mixture and place the egg slices.

Drizzle it with the previously prepared Salad Dressing.

Serve hot.

Nutrition (Per Serving)

Calories: 406

Fat: 22g

Carbohydrates: 28g

Protein: 26g

Wild Rice Soup & Creamy Chicken

Difficulty Level: 2/5

Preparation time: 5 minutes

Cooking time: 15 minutes

Servings: 8

Ingredients

4 cups of chicken broth

2 cups of water

2 half-cooked and boneless chicken breast, grated

1 pack (4.5 ounces) of long-grain fast-cooking rice with a spice pack

1/2 teaspoon of salt

1/2 teaspoon of ground black pepper

3/4 cup flour

1/2 cup butter

2 cups thick cream

Directions:

Combine broth, water, and chicken in a large saucepan over medium heat. Bring to a boil, stir in the rice, and save the seasoning package. Cover and remove from heat.

Combine salt, pepper, and flour in a small bowl. Melt the butter in a medium-sized pan over medium heat. Stir the contents of the herb bag until the mixture bubbles. Reduce the heat and add the flour mixture to the tablespoon to form a roux. Stir the cream little by little until it is completely absorbed and smooth. Bake until thick, 5 minutes.

Add the cream mixture to the stock and rice — Cook over medium heat for 10 to 15 minutes.

Nutrition: (Per Serving)

Per serving:

Calories 462;

Fat 36.5 grams;

Carbohydrates 22.6 g;

Protein 12 g;

Cholesterol 135 mg;

Sodium 997 mg.

Garlic Rice

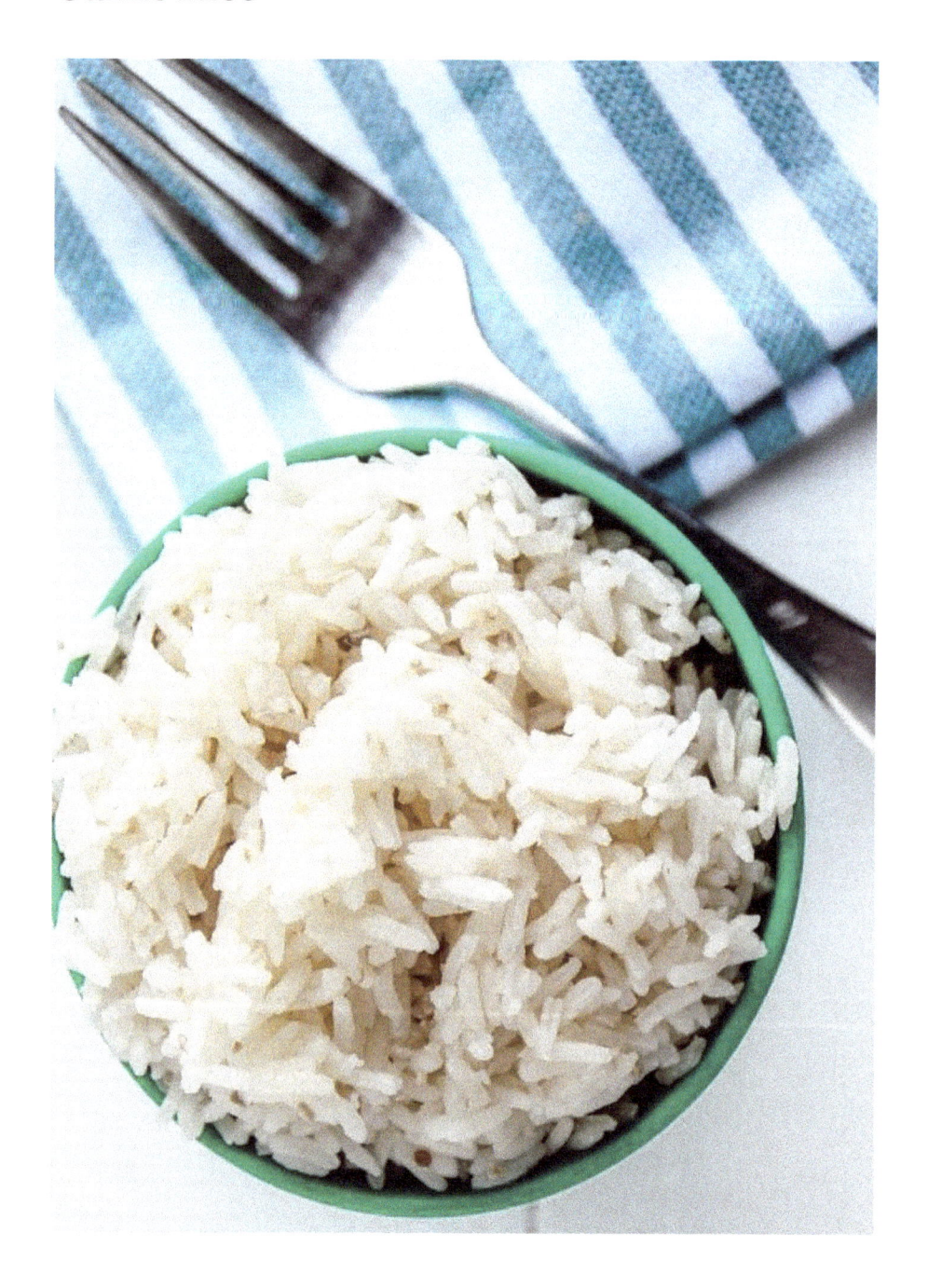

Difficulty Level: 2/5

Preparation time: 5 minutes

Cooking time: 3 minutes

Servings: 4

Ingredients

2 tablespoons vegetable oil

1 1/2 tablespoons chopped garlic

2 tablespoons ground pork

4 cups cooked white rice

1 1/2 teaspoons of garlic salt

ground black pepper to taste

Directions:

Heat the oil in a large frying pan over medium heat. When the oil is hot, add the garlic and ground pork. Boil and stir until garlic is golden brown.

Stir in cooked white rice and season with garlic salt and pepper. Bake and stir until the mixture is hot and well mixed for about 3 minutes.

Nutrition: (Per Serving)

Calories 293;

Fat 9 g;

Carbohydrates 45.9 g;

Protein 5.9 g

Cholesterol 6 mg;

Sodium 686 mg

Carrot Rice

Difficulty Level: 2/5

Preparation time: 5 minutes

Cooking time: 25 minutes

Servings: 6

Ingredients

2 cups of water

1 cube chicken broth

1 grated carrot

1 cup uncooked long-grain rice

Directions:

Bring the water to a boil in a medium-sized saucepan over medium heat. Place in the bouillon cube and let it dissolve.

Stir in the carrots and rice and bring to a boil again.

Lower the heat, cover, and simmer for 20 minutes.

Remove from heat and leave under cover for 5 minutes.

Nutrition: (Per Serving)

Calories 125;

Fat 0.3 g;

Carbohydrates 27.1 g;

Protein 2.7 g;

Cholesterol <1 mg;

Sodium 199 mg.

Pasta Salad with Chicken Club
Difficulty Level: 2/5

Preparation time: 20 minutes

Cooking time: 10 minutes

Servings: 6

Ingredients:

8 oz corkscrew pasta

3/4 cup Italian dressing

1/4 cup mayonnaise

2 cups roasted chicken cooked and minced

12 slices of crispy cooked bacon, crumbled

1 cup diced Münster cheese

1 cup chopped celery

1 cup chopped green pepper

8 oz. Cherry tomatoes, halved

1 avocado - peeled, seeded and chopped

Directions:

Bring a large pan of lightly salted water to a boil. Boil the pasta, occasionally stirring until well-cooked but firm, 10 to 12 minutes. Drain and rinse with cold water.

Beat the Italian dressing and mayonnaise in a large bowl. Stir the pasta, chicken, bacon, Münster cheese, celery, green pepper, cherry tomatoes, and avocado through the vinaigrette until everything is well mixed.

Nutrition: (Per Serving)

485 calories;

30.1 g fat;

37.1 g carbohydrates;

19.2 g of protein;

48 mg cholesterol;

723 mg of sodium.

Tomato Cream Sauce

Difficulty Level: 2/5

Preparation time: 5 minutes

Cooking time: 10 minutes

Servings: 5

Ingredients

2 tablespoons olive oil

1 onion, diced, 1 clove of garlic

1 can diced Italian tomatoes, not drained

1 tablespoon dried basil leaves

3/4 teaspoon white sugar

1/4 teaspoon dried oregano

1/4 teaspoon salt

1/8 teaspoon ground black pepper

1/2 cup heavy cream

1 tablespoon butter

Directions:

Fry onion and garlic in olive oil over medium heat.

Add tomatoes, basil, sugar, oregano, salt and pepper. Bring to a boil and cook for another 5 minutes or until most of the liquid has evaporated.

Remove from the heat; Stir in whipped cream and butter. Reduce the heat and simmer for another 5 minutes.

Nutrition: (Per Serving)

182 calories;

16.6 g fat;

6.7 grams of carbohydrates;

1.7 g of protein;

39 mg cholesterol;

270 mg of sodium.

Alfredo Peppered Shrimp

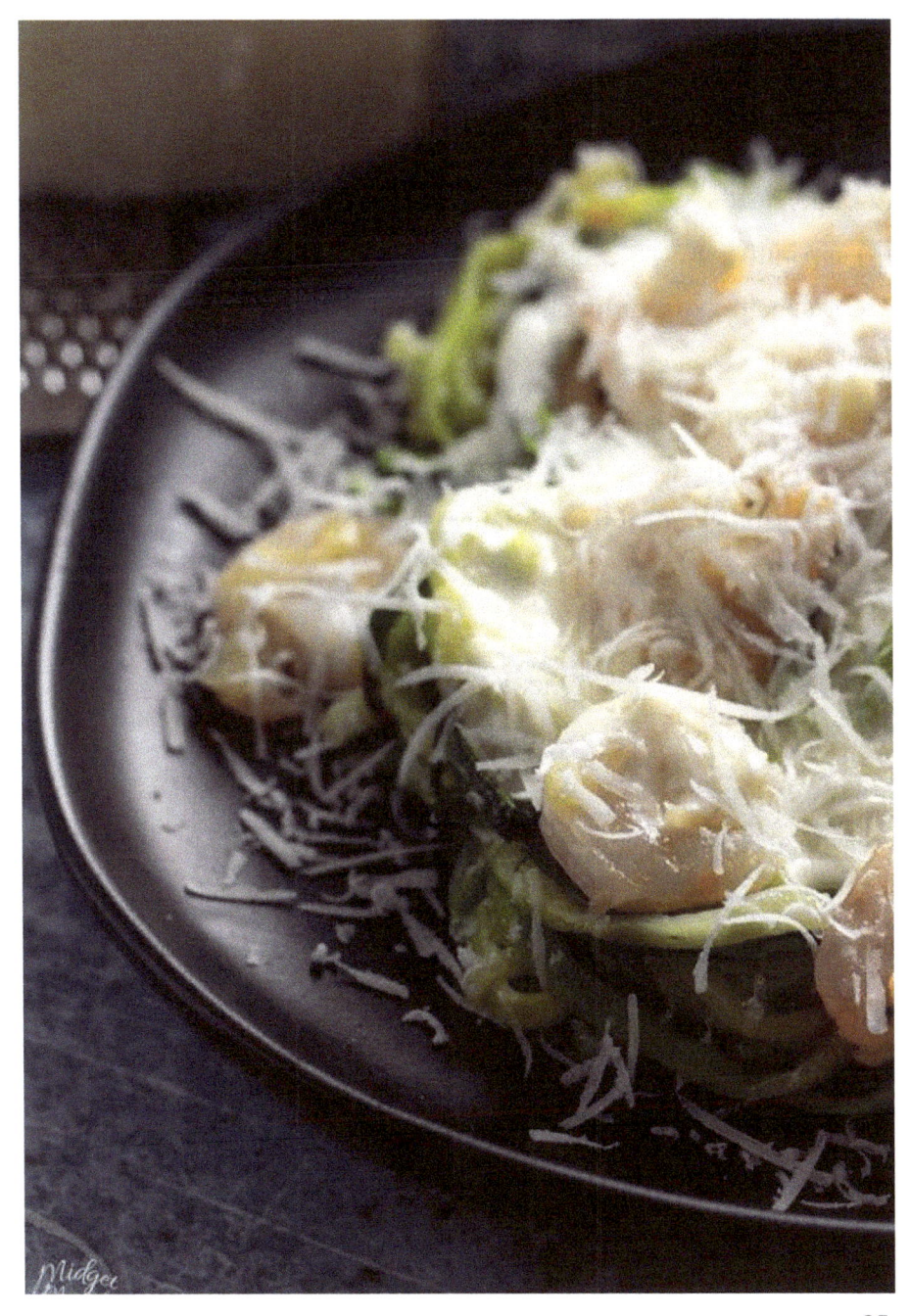

Difficulty Level: 2/5

Preparation time: 5 minutes

Cooking time: 20 minutes

Servings: 6

Ingredients

12 kg penne

1/4 cup butter

2 tablespoons extra virgin olive oil

1 onion, diced

2 cloves of chopped garlic

1 red pepper, diced

1/2 kg Portobello mushrooms, cubed

1 pound shrimp, peeled and thawed

1 jar of Alfredo sauce

1/2 cup of grated Romano cheese

1/2 cup of cream

1/4 cup chopped parsley

1 teaspoon cayenne pepper

salt and pepper to taste

Directions:

Bring a large pot of lightly salted water to a boil. Put the pasta and cook for 8 to 10 minutes or until al dente; drain.

Meanwhile, melt the butter and olive oil in a pan over medium heat. Stir in the onion and cook until soft and translucent, about 2 minutes. Stir in garlic, red pepper and mushrooms; cook over medium heat until soft, about 2 minutes longer.

Stir in the shrimp and fry until firm and pink, then add Alfredo sauce, Romano cheese and cream; bring to a boil, constantly stirring until thick, about 5 minutes. Season with cayenne pepper, salt, and pepper to taste. Add the drained pasta to the sauce and sprinkle with chopped parsley.

Nutrition: (Per Serving)

707 calories;

45 g fat;

50.6 g carbohydrates;

28.4 g of protein;

201 mg of cholesterol;

1034 mg of sodium.

Pesto with Basil and Spinach

Difficulty Level: 2/5

Preparation time: 20 minutes

Cooking time: 0 minutes

Servings: 24

Ingredients

1 1/2 cup small spinach leaves

3/4 cup fresh basil leaves

1/2 cup grilled pine nuts

1/2 cup grated Parmesan cheese

4 cloves of garlic, peeled and quartered

3/4 teaspoon of kosher salt

1/2 teaspoon freshly ground black pepper

1 tablespoon fresh lemon juice

1/2 teaspoon lemon zest

1/2 cup extra virgin olive oil

Directions:

Mix spinach, basil, pine nuts, Parmesan, garlic, salt, pepper, lemon juice, lemon zest, and 2 tablespoons of olive oil in a food processor until smooth.

Sprinkle the remaining olive oil into the mixture.

Nutrition: (Per Serving)

67 calories;

6.6 g fat;

0.8 g carbohydrates;

1.5 g of protein;

1 mg cholesterol;

87 mg of sodium.

Blackened Salmon Fillets

Difficulty Level: 2/5

Preparation time: 15 minutes

Cooking time: 5 minutes

Servings: 4

Ingredients

2 tablespoons paprika powder

1 tablespoon cayenne pepper powder

1 tablespoon onion powder

2 teaspoons salt

1/2 teaspoon ground white pepper

1/2 teaspoon ground black pepper

1/4 teaspoon dried thyme

1/4 teaspoon dried basil

1/4 teaspoon dried oregano

4 salmon fillets, skin and bones removed

1/2 cup unsalted butter, melted

Directions:

Combine bell pepper, cayenne pepper, onion powder, salt, white pepper, black pepper, thyme, basil and oregano in a small bowl.

Brush salmon fillets with 1/4 cup butter and sprinkle evenly with the cayenne pepper mixture. Sprinkle each fillet with ½ of the remaining butter.

Cook the salmon in a large heavy-bottomed pan, until dark, 2 to 5 minutes. Turn the fillets, sprinkle with the remaining butter and continue to cook until the fish easily peels with a fork.

Nutrition: (Per Serving)

511 calories;

38.3 grams of fat;

4.5 grams of carbohydrates

37.4 g of protein;

166 mg cholesterol;

1248 mg of sodium

Mediterranean Baba Ghanoush

Difficulty Level: 3/5

Preparation time: 5 minutes

Cooking time: 25 minutes

Servings: 4

Ingredients:

1 bulb garlic

1 red bell pepper, halved and seeded

1 tbsp chopped fresh basil

1 tbsp olive oil

1 tsp black pepper

2 eggplants, sliced lengthwise

2 rounds of flatbread or pita

Juice of 1 lemon

Directions:

Grease grill grate with cooking spray and preheat grill to medium high.

Slice tops of garlic bulb and wrap in foil. Place in the cooler portion of the grill and roast for at least 20 minutes.

Place bell pepper and eggplant slices on the hottest part of grill.

Grill for at least two to three minutes each side.

Once bulbs are done, peel off skins of roasted garlic and place peeled garlic into food processor.

Add olive oil, pepper, basil, lemon juice, grilled red bell pepper and grilled eggplant.

Puree until smooth and transfer into a bowl.

Grill bread at least 30 seconds per side to warm.

Serve bread with the pureed dip and enjoy.

Nutrition:

Calories: 213.6

Fiber: 36.3g

Carbohydrates: 6.3g

Protein: 4.8g

Tasty Crabby Panini

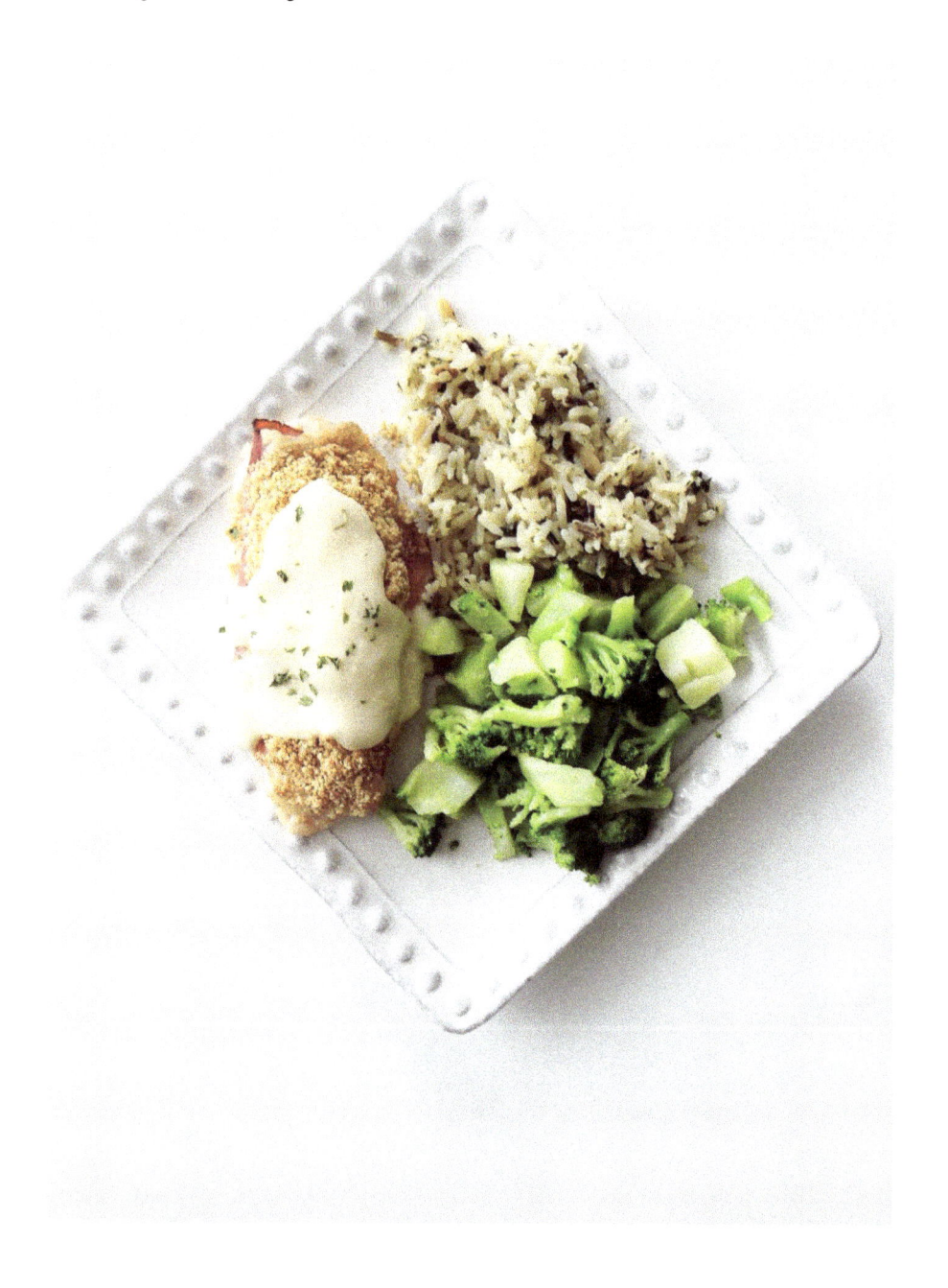

Difficulty Level: 2/5

Preparation time: 10 minutes

Cooking time: 10 minutes

Servings: 4

Ingredients:

1 tbsp Olive oil

French bread split and sliced diagonally

1 lb. blue crab meat or shrimp or spiny lobster or stone crab

½ cup celery

¼ cup green onion chopped

1 tsp Worcestershire sauce

1 tsp lemon juice

1 tbsp Dijon mustard

½ cup light mayonnaise

Directions:

In a medium bowl mix the following thoroughly: celery, onion, Worcestershire, lemon juice, mustard and mayonnaise. Season with pepper and salt. Then gently add in the almonds and crabs.

Spread olive oil on sliced sides of bread and smear with crab mixture before covering with another bread slice.

Grill sandwich in a Panini press until bread is crisped and ridged.

Nutrition:

Calories: 248

Fiber: 10.9g

Carbohydrates: 12.0g

Protein: 24.5g

Bean and Toasted Pita Salad

Difficulty Level: 2/5

Preparation time: 15 minutes

Cooking time: 10 minutes

Servings: 4

Ingredients:

3 tbsp chopped fresh mint

3 tbsp chopped fresh parsley

1 cup crumbled feta cheese

1 cup sliced romaine lettuce

½ cucumber, peeled and sliced

1 cup diced plum tomatoes

2 cups cooked pinto beans, well drained and slightly warmed

Pepper to taste

3 tbsp extra virgin olive oil

2 tbsp ground toasted cumin seeds

2 tbsp fresh lemon juice

1/8 tsp salt

2 cloves garlic, peeled

2 6-inch whole wheat pita bread, cut or torn into bite-sized pieces

Directions:

In large baking sheet, spread torn pita bread and bake in a preheated 400oF oven for 6 minutes.

With the back of a knife, mash garlic and salt until paste like. Add into a medium bowl.

Whisk in ground cumin and lemon juice. In a steady and slow stream, pour oil as you whisk continuously. Season with pepper.

In a large salad bowl, mix cucumber, tomatoes and beans. Pour in dressing, toss to coat well.

Add mint, parsley, feta, lettuce and toasted pita, toss to mix once again and serve.

Nutrition:

Calories: 427

Carbohydrates: 47.3g

Protein: 17.7g

Fat: 20.4g

Goat Cheese 'n Red Beans Salad

Difficulty Level: 1/5

Preparation time: 15 minutes

Cooking time: 0 minutes

Servings: 4

Ingredients:

2 cans of Red Kidney Beans, drained and rinsed well

Water or vegetable broth to cover beans

1 bunch parsley, chopped

1 1/2 cups red grape tomatoes, halved

3 cloves garlic, minced

3 tablespoons olive oil

3 tablespoons lemon juice

1/2 teaspoon salt

1/2 teaspoon white pepper

6 ounces goat cheese, crumbled

Directions:

In a large bowl, combine beans, parsley, tomatoes and garlic.

Add olive oil, lemon juice, salt and pepper.

Mix well and refrigerate until ready to serve.

Spoon into individual dishes topped with crumbled goat cheese.

Nutrition:

Calories: 385

Carbohydrates: 44.0g

Protein: 22.5g

Fat: 15.0g

Spicy Sweet Red Hummus

Difficulty Level: 1/5

Preparation time: 10 minutes

Cooking time: 0 minutes

Servings: 8

Ingredients:

1 (15 ounce) can garbanzo beans, drained

1 (4 ounce) jar roasted red peppers

1 1/2 tablespoons tahini

1 clove garlic, minced

1 tablespoon chopped fresh parsley

1/2 teaspoon cayenne pepper

1/2 teaspoon ground cumin

1/4 teaspoon salt

3 tablespoons lemon juice

Directions:

In a blender, add all ingredients and process until smooth and creamy.

Adjust seasoning to taste if needed.

Can be stored in an airtight container for up to 5 days.

Nutrition:

Calories: 64

Carbohydrates: 9.6g

Protein: 2.5g

Fat: 2.2g

Dill Relish on White Sea Bass

Difficulty Level: 2/5

Preparation time: 15 minutes

Cooking time: 12 minutes

Servings: 4

Ingredients:

1 ½ tbsp chopped white onion

1 ½ tsp chopped fresh dill

1 lemon, quartered

1 tsp Dijon mustard

1 tsp lemon juice

1 tsp pickled baby capers, drained

4 pieces of 4-oz white sea bass fillets

Directions:

Preheat oven to 375oF.

Mix lemon juice, mustard, dill, capers and onions in a small bowl.

Prepare four aluminum foil squares and place 1 fillet per foil.

Squeeze a lemon wedge per fish.

Evenly divide into 4 the dill spread and drizzle over fillet.

Close the foil over the fish securely and pop in the oven.

Bake for 10 to 12 minutes or until fish is cooked through.

Remove from foil and transfer to a serving platter, serve and enjoy.

Nutrition:

Calories: 115

Carbohydrates: 12g

Protein: 7g

Fat: 1g

Vegetable Lover's Chicken Soup

Difficulty Level: 2/5

Preparation time: 10 minutes

Cooking time: 20 minutes

Servings: 4

Ingredients:

1 ½ cups baby spinach

2 tbsp orzo (tiny pasta)

¼ cup dry white wine

1 14oz low sodium chicken broth

2 plum tomatoes, chopped

1/8 tsp salt

½ tsp Italian seasoning

1 large shallot, chopped

1 small zucchini, diced

8-oz chicken tenders

1 tbsp extra virgin olive oil

Directions:

In a large saucepan, heat oil over medium heat and add the chicken. Stir occasionally for 8 minutes until browned. Transfer in a plate. Set aside.

In the same saucepan, add the zucchini, Italian seasoning, shallot and salt and stir often until the vegetables are softened, around 4 minutes.

Add the tomatoes, wine, broth and orzo and increase the heat to high to bring the mixture to boil. Reduce the heat and simmer.

Add the cooked chicken and stir in the spinach last.

Serve hot.

Nutrition:

Calories: 207

Carbohydrates: 14.8g

Protein: 12.2g

Fat: 11.4g

Mustard Chops with Apricot-basil Relish

Difficulty Level: 2/5

Preparation time: 18 minutes

Cooking time: 12 minutes

Servings: 4

Ingredients:

¼ cup basil, finely shredded

¼ cup olive oil

½ cup mustard

¾ lb. fresh apricots, stone removed, and fruit diced

1 shallot, diced small

1 tsp ground cardamom

3 tbsp raspberry vinegar

4 pork chops

Pepper and salt

Directions:

Make sure that pork chops are defrosted well. Season with pepper and salt. Slather both sides of each pork chop with mustard. Preheat grill to medium-high fire.

In a medium bowl, mix cardamom, olive oil, vinegar, basil, shallot, and apricots. Toss to combine and season with pepper and salt, mixing once again.

Grill chops for 5 to 6 minutes per side. As you flip, baste with mustard.

Serve pork chops with the Apricot-Basil relish and enjoy.

Nutrition:

Calories: 486.5

Carbohydrates: 7.3g

Protein: 42.1g

Fat: 32.1g

Seafood and Veggie Pasta

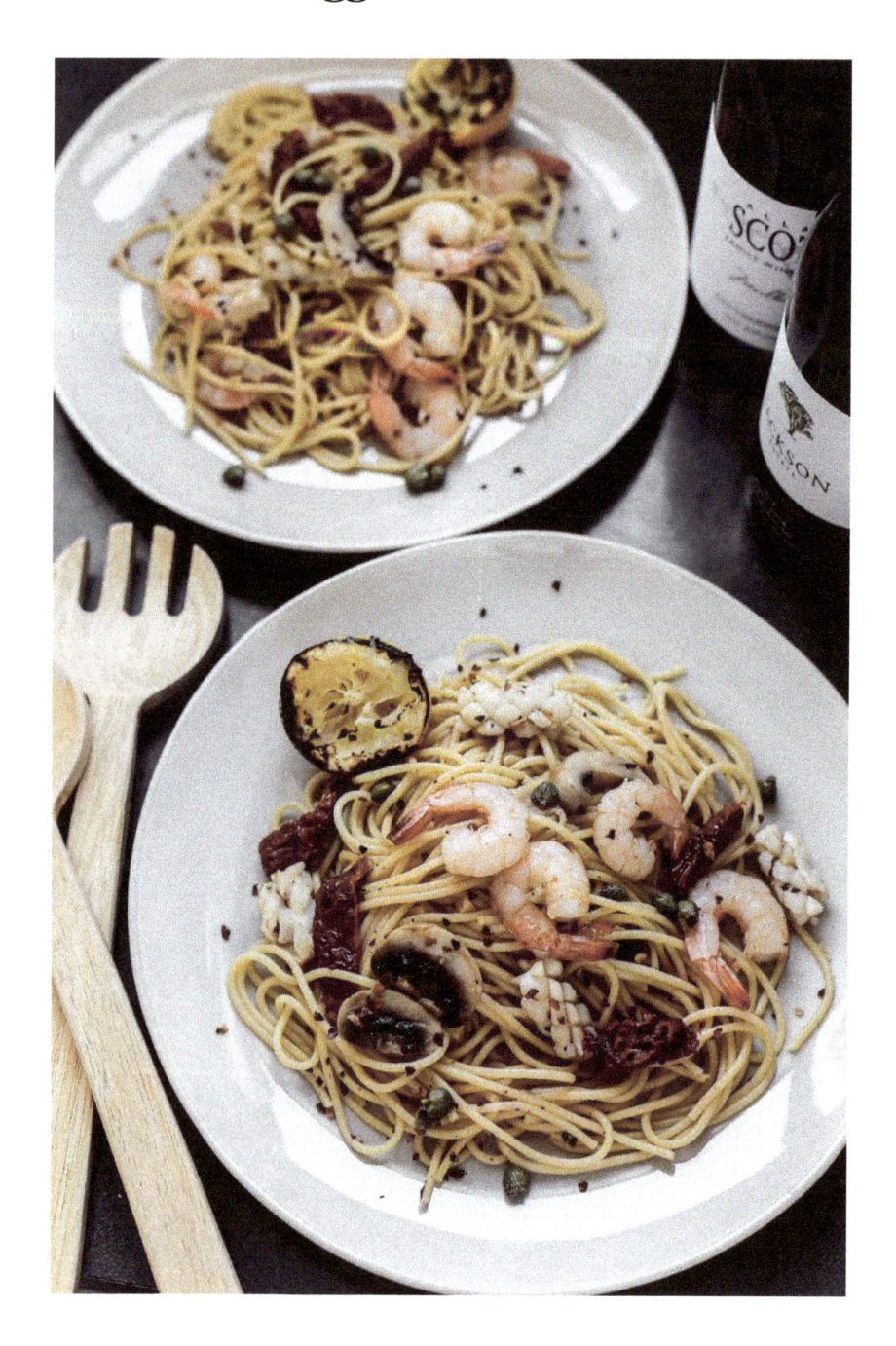

Difficulty Level: 3/5

Preparation time: 10 minutes

Cooking time: 20 minutes

Servings: 4

Ingredients:

¼ tsp pepper

¼ tsp salt

1 lb raw shelled shrimp

1 lemon, cut into wedges

1 tbsp butter

1 tbsp olive oil

2 5-oz cans chopped clams, drained (reserve 2 tbsp clam juice)

2 tbsp dry white wine

4 cloves garlic, minced

4 cups zucchini, spiraled (use a veggie spiralizer)

4 tbsp Parmesan Cheese

Chopped fresh parsley to garnish

Directions:

Ready the zucchini and spiralize with a veggie spiralizer. Arrange 1 cup of zucchini noodle per bowl. Total of 4 bowls.

On medium fire, place a large nonstick saucepan and heat oil and butter.

For a minute, sauté garlic. Add shrimp and cook for 3 minutes until opaque or cooked.

Add white wine, reserved clam juice and clams. Bring to a simmer and continue simmering for 2 minutes or until half of liquid has evaporated. Stir constantly.

Season with pepper and salt. And if needed add more to taste.

Remove from fire and evenly distribute seafood sauce to 4 bowls.

Top with a tablespoonful of Parmesan cheese per bowl, serve and enjoy.

Nutrition:

Calories: 324.9

Carbohydrates: 12g

Protein: 43.8g

Fat: 11.3g

Creamy Alfredo Fettuccine

Difficulty Level: 2/5

Preparation time: 5 minutes

Cooking time: 25 minutes

Servings: 4

Ingredients:

Grated parmesan cheese

½ cup freshly grated parmesan cheese

1/8 tsp freshly ground black pepper

½ tsp salt

1 cup whipping cream

2 tbsp butter

8 oz dried fettuccine, cooked and drained

Directions:

On medium high fire, place a big fry pan and heat butter.

Add pepper, salt and cream and gently boil for three to five minutes.

Once thickened, turn off fire and quickly stir in ½ cup of parmesan cheese. Toss in pasta, mix well.

Top with another batch of parmesan cheese and serve.

Nutrition:

Calories: 202

Carbohydrates: 21.1g

Protein: 7.9g

Fat: 10.2g

Tasty Lasagna Rolls

Difficulty Level: 2/5

Preparation time: 10 minutes

Cooking time: 20 minutes

Servings: 6

Ingredients:

¼ tsp crushed red pepper

¼ tsp salt

½ cup shredded mozzarella cheese

½ cups parmesan cheese, shredded

1 14-oz package tofu, cubed

1 25-oz can of low-sodium marinara sauce

1 tbsp extra virgin olive oil

12 whole wheat lasagna noodles

2 tbsp Kalamata olives, chopped

3 cloves minced garlic

3 cups spinach, chopped

Directions:

Put enough water on a large pot and cook the lasagna noodles according to package instructions. Drain, rinse and set aside until ready to use.

In a large skillet, sauté garlic over medium heat for 20 seconds. Add the tofu and spinach and cook until the spinach wilts. Transfer this mixture in a bowl and add parmesan olives, salt, red pepper and 2/3 cup of the marinara sauce.

In a pan, spread a cup of marinara sauce on the bottom. To make the rolls, place noodle on a surface and spread ¼ cup of the tofu filling. Roll up and place it on the pan with the marinara sauce. Do this procedure until all lasagna noodles are rolled.

Place the pan over high heat and bring to a simmer. Reduce the heat to medium and let it cook for three more minutes. Sprinkle mozzarella cheese and let the cheese melt for two minutes. Serve hot.

Nutrition:

Calories: 304

Carbohydrates: 39.2g

Protein: 23g

Fat: 19.2g

Tortellini Salad with Broccoli

Difficulty Level: 2/5

Preparation time: 10 minutes

Cooking time: 20 minutes

Servings: 12

Ingredients:

1 red onion, chopped finely

1 cup sunflower seeds

1 cup raisins

3 heads fresh broccoli, cut into florets

2 tsp cider vinegar

½ cup white sugar

½ cup mayonnaise

20-oz fresh cheese filled tortellini

Directions:

In a large pot of boiling water, cook tortellini according to manufacturer's instructions. Drain and rinse with cold water and set aside.

Whisk vinegar, sugar and mayonnaise to create your salad dressing.

Mix together in a large bowl red onion, sunflower seeds, raisins, tortellini and broccoli. Pour dressing and toss to coat.

Serve and enjoy.

Nutrition:

Calories: 272

Carbohydrates: 38.7g

Protein: 5.0g

Fat: 8.1g

Simple Penne Anti-Pasto

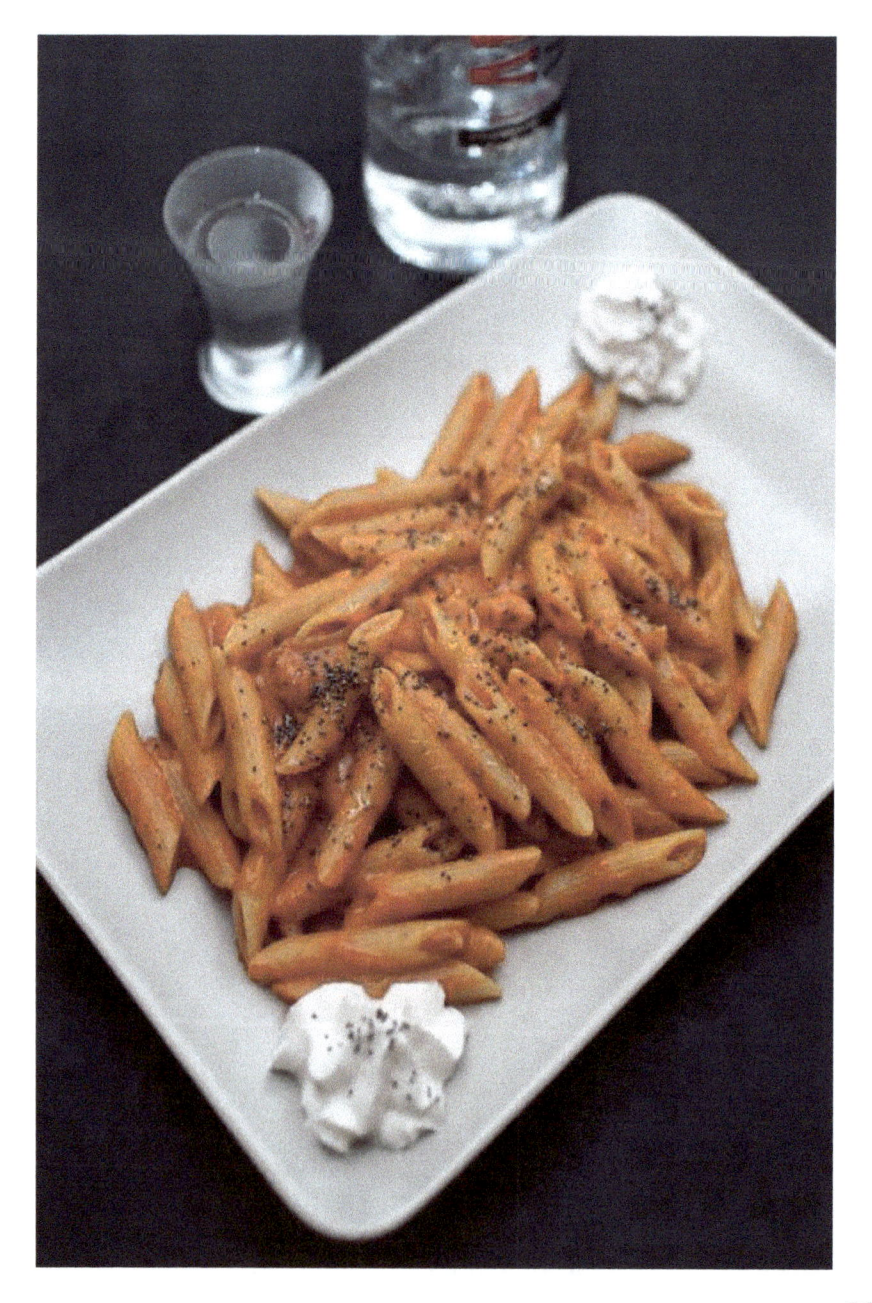

Difficulty Level: 2/5

Preparation time: 15 minutes

Cooking time: 15 minutes

Servings: 4

Ingredients:

¼ cup pine nuts, toasted

½ cup grated Parmigiano-Reggiano cheese, divided

8oz penne pasta, cooked and drained

1 6oz jar drained, sliced, marinated and quartered artichoke hearts

1 7 oz jar drained and chopped sun-dried tomato halves packed in oil

3 oz chopped prosciutto

1/3 cup pesto

½ cup pitted and chopped Kalamata olives

1 medium red bell pepper

Directions:

Slice bell pepper, discard membranes, seeds and stem. On a foiled lined baking sheet, place bell pepper halves, press down by hand and broil in oven for eight minutes. Remove from oven, put in a sealed bag for 5 minutes before peeling and chopping.

Place chopped bell pepper in a bowl and mix in artichokes, tomatoes, prosciutto, pesto and olives.

Toss in ¼ cup cheese and pasta. Transfer to a serving dish and garnish with ¼ cup cheese and pine nuts. Serve and enjoy!

Nutrition:

Calories: 606

Carbohydrates: 70.3g

Protein: 27.2g

Fat: 27.6g

Butternut Squash Hummus

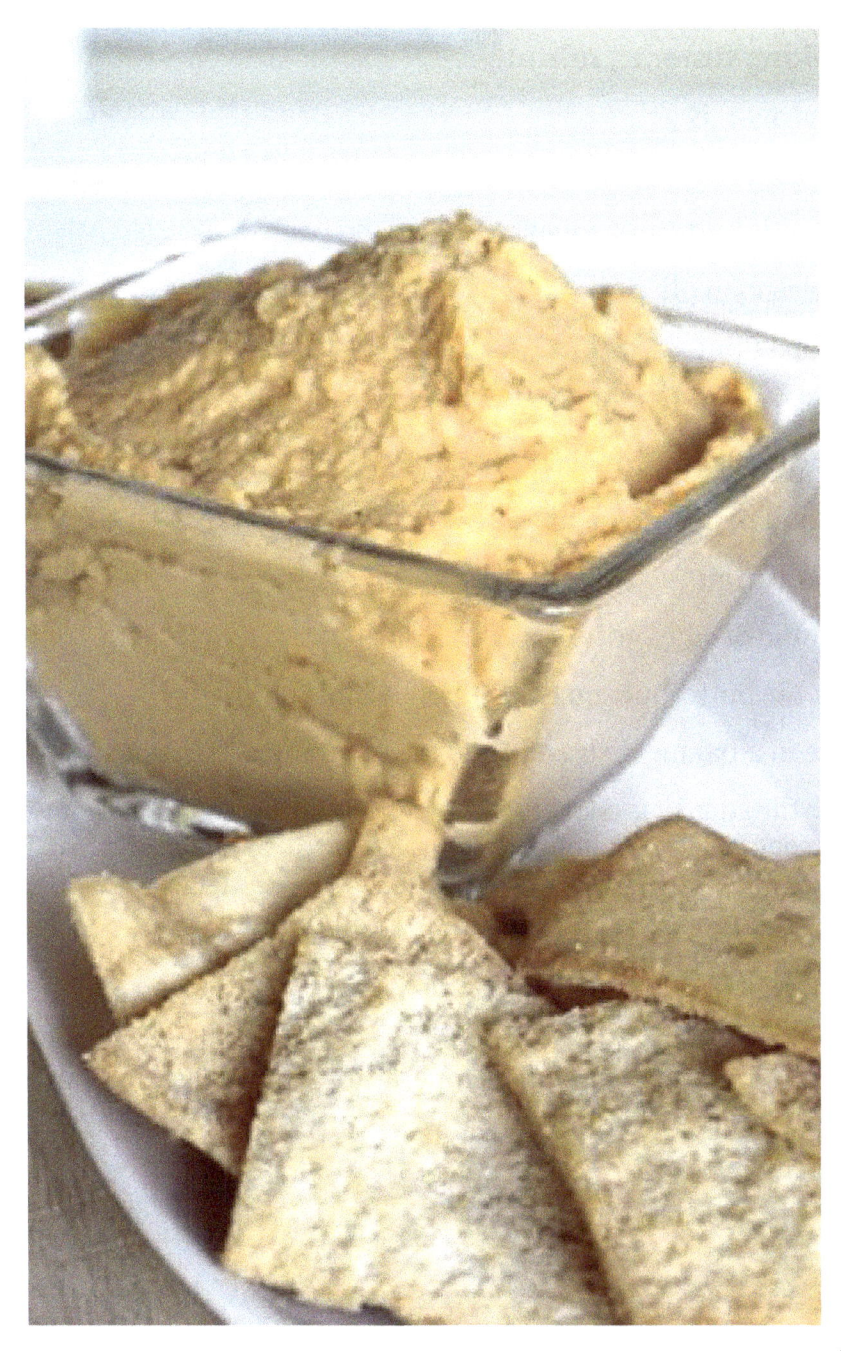

Difficulty Level: 2/5

Preparation time: 15 minutes

Cooking time: 15 minutes

Servings: 8

Ingredients:

2 pounds butternut squash, seeded and peeled

1 tablespoon olive oil

¼ cup tahini

2 tablespoons lemon juice

2 cloves of garlic, minced

Salt and pepper to taste

Directions:

Heat the oven to 300oF.

Coat the butternut squash with olive oil.

Place in a baking dish and bake for 15 minutes in the oven.

Once the squash is cooked, place in a food processor together with the rest of the ingredients.

Pulse until smooth.

Place in individual containers.

Put a label and store in the fridge.

Allow to warm at room temperature before heating in the microwave oven.

Serve with carrots or celery sticks.

Nutrition:

Calories: 115

Carbohydrates: 15.8g

Protein: 2.5g

Fat: 5.8g

Fiber: 6.7g

Parmesan Mashed Potatoes with Olive Oil, Garlic, & Parsley

Difficulty Level: 2/5

Preparation time: 5 minutes

Cooking time: 30 minutes

Servings: 4

Ingredients:

5 pounds red skinned potatoes (chopped into 2 inch pieces)

2 heads roasted garlic

4 tablespoons garlic powder

3 cups heavy cream

1/2 pound Parmesan cheese

1/4 cup fresh parsley (chopped)

1/4 cup olive oil (Pompeian, I love the Mediterranean blend!)

pepper

salt

olive oil (additional, to drizzle & fresh chopped parsley to garnish, optional)

Directions:

Boil the potatoes in enough water to cover until fork tender. Drain. Place the potatoes back into the pot on medium, and mash best you can with a potato masher to release the steam. Pour in the heavy cream, & finish mashing the potatoes. Stir the mixture to combine. Stir in the Parmesan cheese, garlic, & fresh chopped parsley. Drizzle in the olive oil, a little at a time - stirring after each drizzle, until all the olive oil is combined. Season with salt & pepper to taste.

Scoop into your serving vessel; drizzle with olive oil and sprinkle on chopped parsley to garnish if desired

Nutrition: (Per serving)

1570 Calories;

0.113g fat;

0.109g carbs;

0.38g protein;

Greek Cauliflower Rice with Feta and Olives

Difficulty Level: 2/5

Preparation time: 5 minutes

Cooking time: 30 minutes

Servings: 4

Ingredients:

1 shallot (large, diced)

1 tablespoon coconut oil

1 pound cauliflower (aged or shredded in food processor, you can buy it pre-shredded at Trader Joe's in the products section)

1 cup of crumbled feta cheese

1/2 cup sliced black olives (kalamata is great, but every black olive does with it)

1/3 cup parsley (finely chopped, plus more for garnish)

salt

pepper

Directions:

Heat coconut oil in a frying pan over medium heat. When the oil sparkles, add the diced shallot. Sauté until transparent.

Put the cauliflower rice in the pan. Cook for 10-15 minutes, stirring occasionally. Brown the cauliflower a little and then remove from the heat. Stir in the parsley, olives and feta and season with salt and pepper. Garnish with extra parsley if desired. Serve hot.

Nutrition: (Per serving)

200 Calories;

0.13g fat;

0.15g carbs;

0.9g protein

Brussels Sprouts
Difficulty Level: 2/5

Preparation time: 5 minutes

Cooking time: 15 minutes

Servings: 5

Ingredients:

1 pound brussels sprouts (quartered)

1 tablespoon olive oil

1/2 oregano teaspoon

1 teaspoon crushed garlic

1/2 teaspoon of salt

1/4 teaspoon pepper

20 kalamata olives (pitted and halved)

8 sun dried tomatoes (sliced)

1/2 cup of feta cheese

1/2 cup sliced almonds (toasted)

Directions:

Cook Brussels in the microwave for 4 minutes.

Meanwhile, heat the olive oil and garlic in a large frying pan. Cook for a minute or two.

Add tomatoes, Brussels, olives, oregano, salt and pepper.

Bake for a few minutes.

In the meantime, roast for a few minutes in a dry frying pan. Be careful not to burn them.

When almonds are a little roasted. Remove everything from the stove.

1. Add the feta cheese and sprinkle the almonds on top and serve.

Nutrition: (Per serving)

180 Calories;

0.1g fat;

0.14g carbs;

0.8g protein

Garlic Scapes Sautéed with Olive Oil, Sea Salt & Freshly Ground Pepper

Difficulty Level: 2/5

Preparation time: 5 minutes

Cooking time: 25 minutes

Servings: 2

Ingredients:

1 bunch of garlic scapes (about 12 to 14 votes)

1 olive oil teaspoon

sea salt (to taste, I use Mediterranean sea salt)

freshly ground black pepper (to taste)

Directions:

Rinse garlic scapes under cold water in a colander. Cut off the hard lower part of the vote. Pat dry.

Add olive to a flat wide pan over medium high heat, heat for about a minute. Add the garlic scapes, sprinkle with salt and freshly ground pepper. Sauté for about a minute, flip the scapes over and fry on the other side.

Add about a teaspoon of water, cover the pan with a fitted member and let it steam for a few minutes until tender. Lift the member and check for done-ness. If the scapes are getting too dry but are not tender yet, add another spoon of water, cover and steam.

When the stems are tender (check with a fork), uncover and fry for another minute. Scapes should be lightly charred, they're tastier that way. Remove from heat and serve immediately.

Nutrition: (Per serving)

Calories: 301;

Protein: 17g;

Total Carbohydrates: 29g;

Sugars: 2g;

Fiber: 17g;

Total Fat: 14g;

Saturated Fat: 2g;

Julene's Green Juice

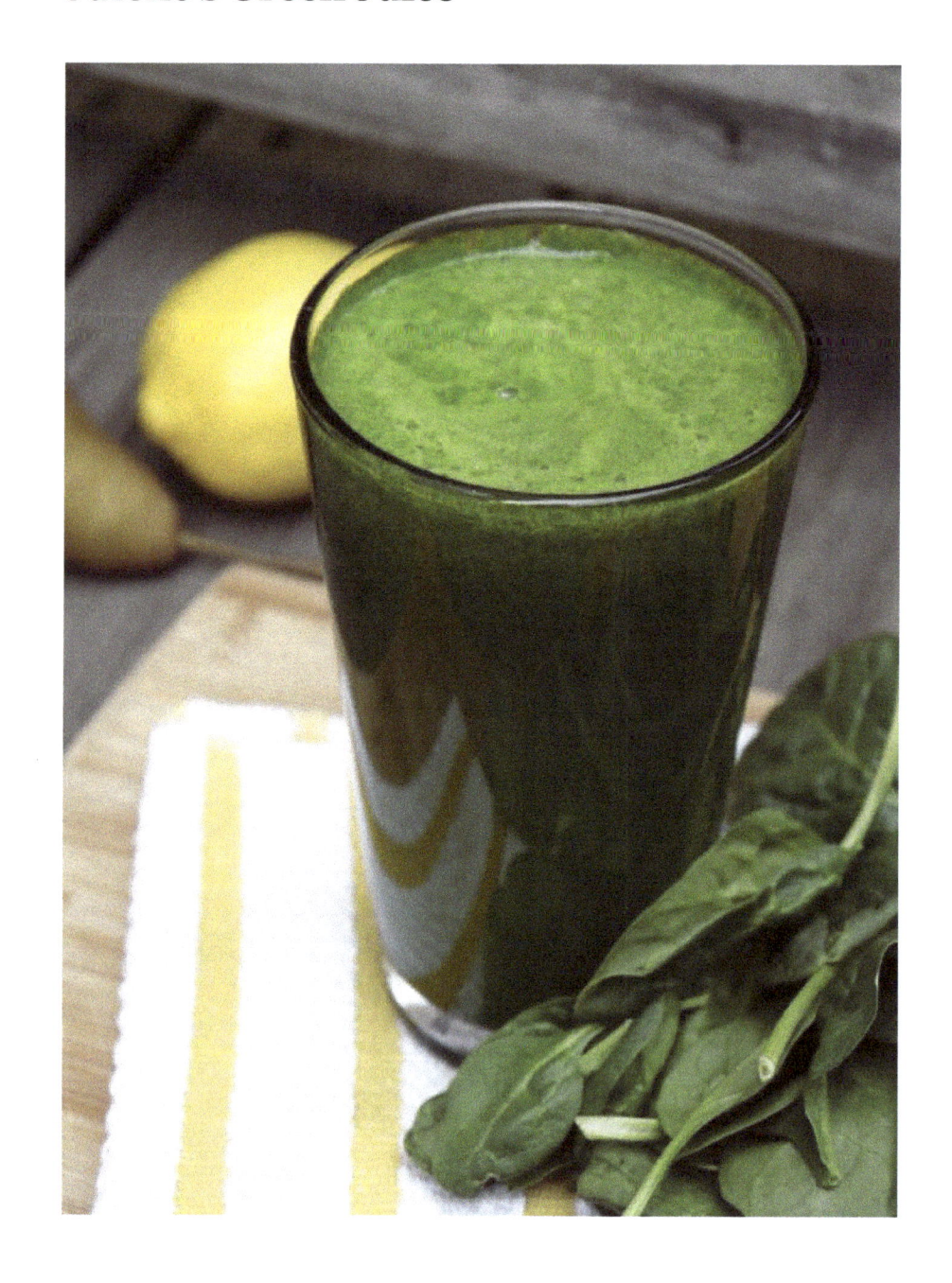

Difficulty Level: 1/5

Preparation time: 5 minutes

Cooking time: 0 minutes

Servings: 1

Ingredients:

3 cups dark leafy greens

1 cucumber

¼ cup fresh Italian parsley leaves

¼ pineapple, cut into wedges

½ green apple

½ orange

½ lemon

Pinch grated fresh ginger

Directions:

Using a juicer, run the greens, cucumber, parsley, pineapple, apple, orange, lemon, and ginger through it, pour into a large cup, and serve.

Nutrition:

Calories: 108;

Protein: 11g;

Carbohydrates: 29g;

Sugars: 10g;

Fiber: 9g;

Total Fat: 2g;

Saturated Fat: 0g;

Cholesterol: 0mg;
Sodium: 119mg

Chocolate Banana Smoothie

Difficulty Level: 1/5

Preparation time: 5 minutes

Cooking time: 0 minutes

Servings: 2

Ingredients:

2 bananas, peeled

1 cup unsweetened almond milk, or skim milk

1 cup crushed ice

3 tablespoons unsweetened cocoa powder

3 tablespoons honey

Directions:

In a blender, combine the bananas, almond milk, ice, cocoa powder, and honey. Blend until smooth.

Nutrition:

Calories: 219;

Protein: 2g;

Total Carbohydrates: 57g;

Sugars: 40g;

Fiber: 6g;

Total Fat: 2g;

Saturated Fat: <1g;

Cholesterol: 0mg;

Sodium: 4mg

Fruit Smoothie

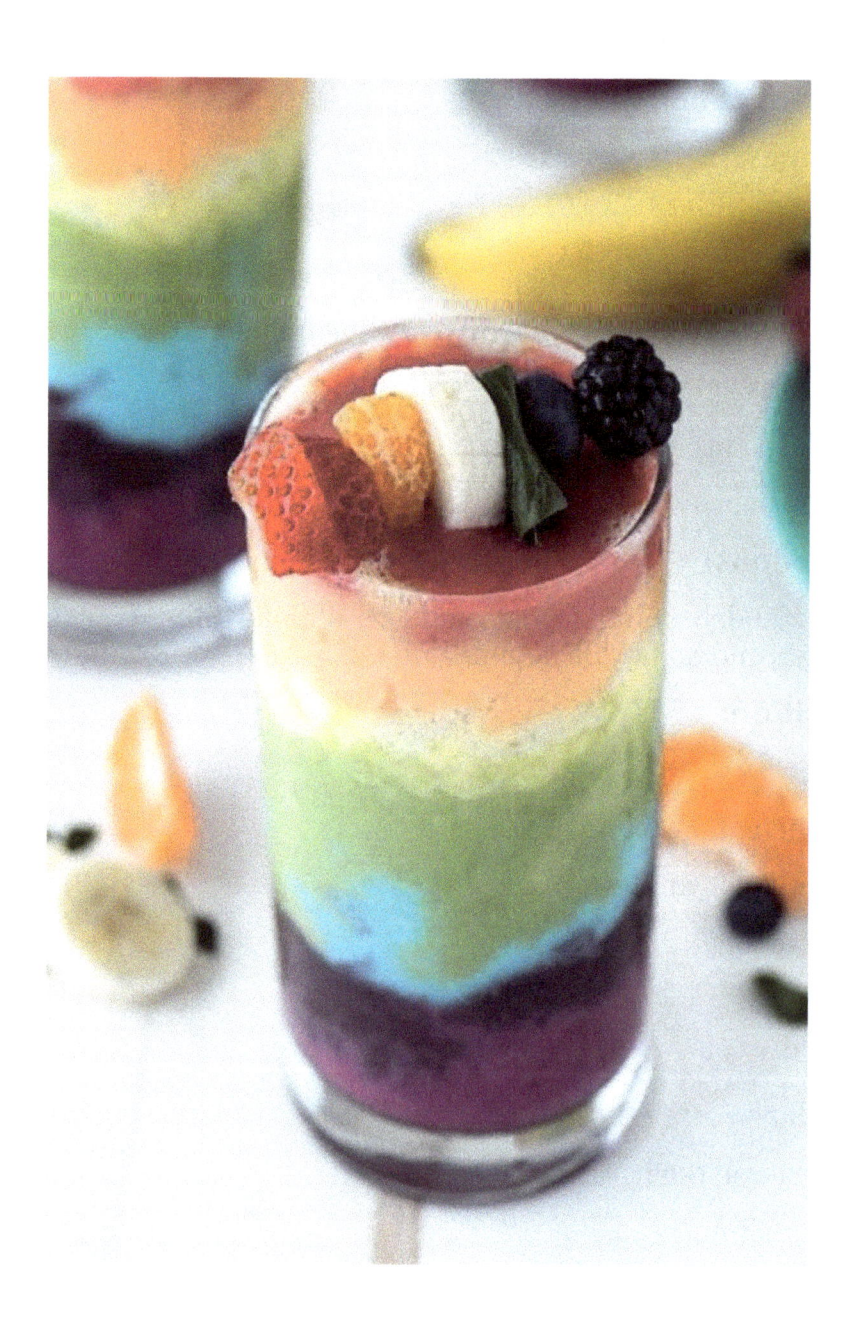

Difficulty Level: 1/5

Preparation time: 5 minutes

Cooking time: 0 minutes

Servings: 2

Ingredients:

2 cups blueberries (or any fresh or frozen fruit, cut into pieces if the fruit is large)

2 cups unsweetened almond milk

1 cup crushed ice

½ teaspoon ground ginger (or other dried ground spice such as turmeric, cinnamon, or nutmeg)

Directions:

In a blender, combine the blueberries, almond milk, ice, and ginger. Blend until smooth.

Nutrition:

Calories: 125;

Protein: 2g;

Total Carbohydrates: 23g;

Sugars: 14g;

Fiber: 5g;

Total Fat: 4g;

Fat: <1g;

Cholesterol: 0mg;

Sodium: 181mg

Chia-Pomegranate Smoothie

Difficulty Level: 2/5

Preparation time: 5 minutes

Cooking time: 0 minutes

Servings: 2

Ingredients:

1 cup pure pomegranate juice (no sugar added)

1 cup frozen berries

1 cup coarsely chopped kale

2 tablespoons chia seeds

3 Medjool dates, pitted and coarsely chopped

Pinch ground cinnamon

Directions:

In a blender, combine the pomegranate juice, berries, kale, chia seeds, dates, and cinnamon and pulse until smooth. Pour into glasses and serve.

Nutrition:

Calories: 275;

Total fat: 5g;

Saturated fat: 1g;

Carbohydrates: 59g;

Sugar: 10g;

Fiber: 42g;

Protein: 5g

Sweet Kale Smoothie

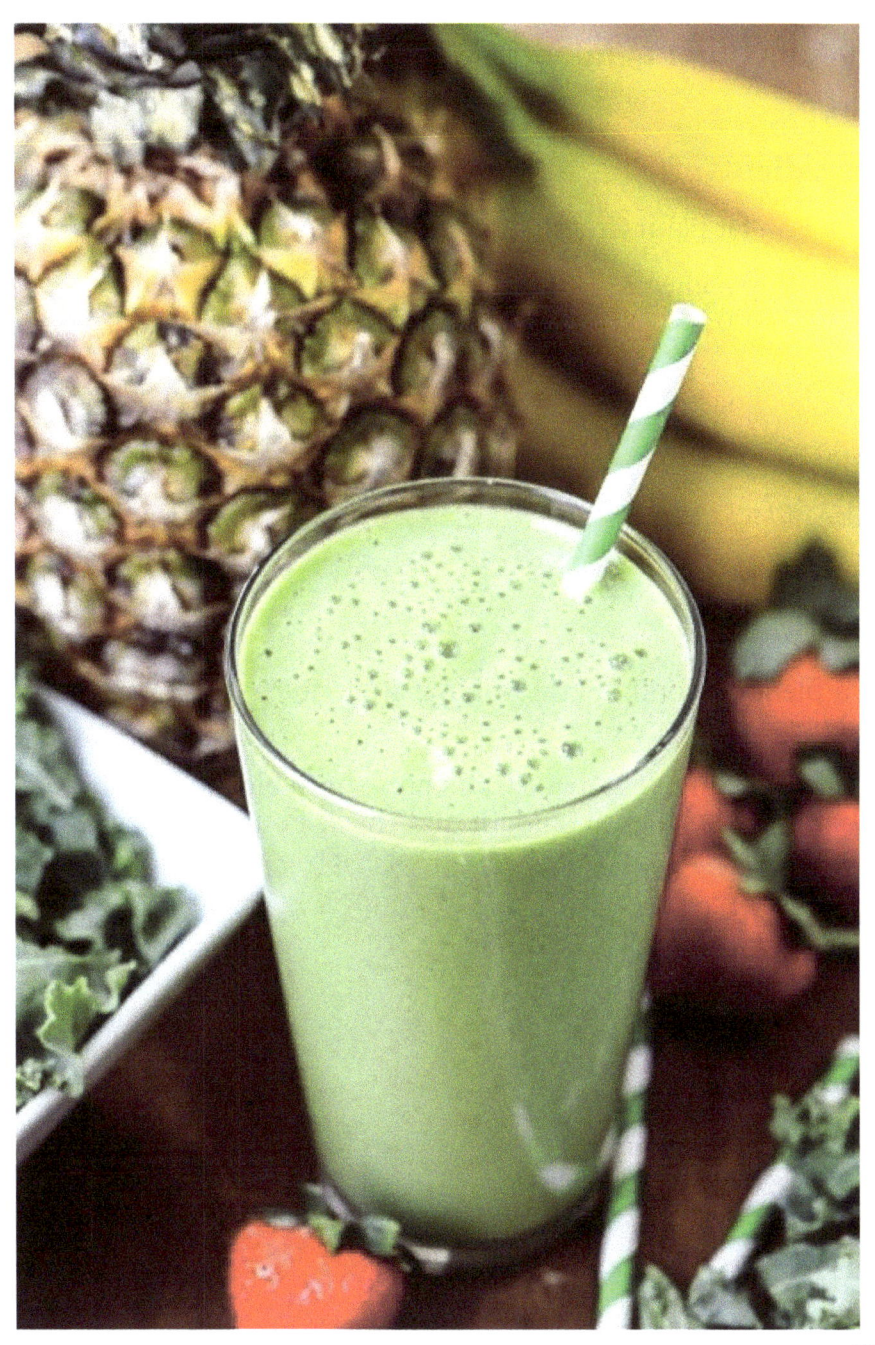

Difficulty Level: 2/5

Preparation time: 10 minutes

Cooking time: 15 minutes

Servings: 2

Ingredients:

1 cup low-fat plain Greek yogurt

½ cup apple juice

1 apple, cored and quartered

4 Medjool dates

3 cups packed coarsely chopped kale

Juice of ½ lemon

4 ice cubes

Directions:

In a blender, combine the yogurt, apple juice, apple, and dates and pulse until smooth.

Add the kale and lemon juice and pulse until blended. Add the ice cubes and blend until smooth and thick. Pour into glasses and serve.

Nutrition:

Calories: 355;

Total fat: 2g;

Saturated fat: 1g;

Carbohydrates: 77g;

Sugar: 58g;

Fiber: 8g;

Protein: 11g

Avocado-Blueberry Smoothie

Difficulty Level: 2/5

Preparation time: 5 minutes

Cooking time: 0 minutes

Servings: 2

Ingredients:

½ cup unsweetened vanilla almond milk

½ cup low-fat plain Greek yogurt

1 ripe avocado, peeled, pitted, and coarsely chopped

1 cup blueberries

¼ cup gluten-free rolled oats

½ teaspoon vanilla extract

4 ice cubes

Directions:

In a blender, combine the almond milk, yogurt, avocado, blueberries, oats, and vanilla and pulse until well blended.

Add the ice cubes and blend until thick and smooth. Serve.

Nutrition:

Calories: 273;

Total fat: 15g;

Saturated fat: 2g;

Carbohydrates: 28g;

Sugar: 10g;

Fiber: 9g;

Protein: 10g

Cranberry-Pumpkin Smoothie

Difficulty Level: 2/5

Preparation time: 5 minutes

Cooking time: 0 minutes

Servings: 2

Ingredients:

2 cups unsweetened almond milk

1 cup pure pumpkin purée

¼ cup gluten-free rolled oats

¼ cup pure cranberry juice (no sugar added)

1 tablespoon honey

¼ teaspoon ground cinnamon

Pinch ground nutmeg

Directions:

In a blender, combine the almond milk, pumpkin, oats, cranberry juice, honey, cinnamon, and nutmeg and blend until smooth.

Pour into glasses and serve immediately.

Nutrition:

Calories: 190;

Total fat: 7g;

Saturated fat: 0g;

Carbohydrates: 26g;

Sugar: 12g;

Fiber: 5g;

Protein: 4g

Sweet Cranberry Nectar

Preparation time: 8 minutes

Cooking time: 5 minutes

Servings: 4

Ingredients:

4 cups fresh cranberries

1 fresh lemon juice

½ cup agave nectar

1 piece of cinnamon stick

1-gallon water, filtered

Directions:

Add cranberries, ½ gallon water, and cinnamon into your pot

Close the lid

Cook on HIGH pressure for 8 minutes

Release the pressure naturally

Firstly, strain the liquid, then add remaining water

Cool, add agave nectar and lemon

Served chill and enjoy!

Nutrition (Per Serving)

Calories: 184

Fat: 0g

Carbohydrates: 49g

Protein: 1g

Hearty Pear and Mango Smoothie
Difficulty Level: 2/5

Preparation time: 10 minutes

Cooking time: nil

Servings: 1

Ingredients:

1 ripe mango, cored and chopped

½ mango, peeled, pitted and chopped

1 cup kale, chopped

½ cup plain Greek yogurt

2 ice cubes

Directions:

Add pear, mango, yogurt, kale, and mango to a blender and puree.

Add ice and blend until you have a smooth texture.

Serve and enjoy!

Nutrition (Per Serving)

Calories: 293

Fat: 8g

Carbohydrates: 53g

Protein: 8g

Fig Smoothie with Cinnamon

Difficulty Level: 2/5

Preparation time: 5 minutes

Cooking time: 10 minutes

Servings: 2

Ingredients:

3 dessertspoons porridge oats

1 large ripe fig

6 ¾ oz. orange juice

3 rounded dessertspoons Greek yogurt

½ teaspoon ground cinnamon

3 ice cubes

Directions:

Wash and dry the fig and chop roughly. Reserve some for topping.

Add all ingredients to a blender, except for the ice cubes.

Add a little water to thin the smoothie and add an ice cube at the end.

Top with some cinnamon, a teaspoon of yogurt, and reserved fig. Finally, serve.

Nutrition (per serving):

Calories 92;

Fat 1.1 g;

Carbohydrates 20 g total;

Protein 3 g

Breakfast Almond Milk Shake

Preparation Time: 4 minutes

Servings: 2

Ingredients

3 cups almond milk

4 tbsp heavy cream

½ tsp vanilla extract

4 tbsp flax meal

2 tbsp protein powder

4 drops of liquid stevia Ice cubes to serve

Directions

In the bowl of your food processor, add almond milk, heavy cream, flax meal, vanilla extract, collagen peptides, and stevia.

Blitz until uniform and smooth, for about 30 seconds.

Add a bit more almond milk if it's very thick.

Pour in a smoothie glass, add the ice cubes and sprinkle with cinnamon.

Nutrition:

Calories 326,

Fat: 27g;

Net Carbs: 6g;

Protein: 19g

Raspberry Vanilla Smoothie

Difficulty Level: 2/5

Preparation time: 5 minutes

Cooking time: 5 minutes

Servings: over 2 cups

Ingredients:

1 cup frozen raspberries

6-ounce container of vanilla Greek yogurt

½ cup of unsweetened vanilla almond milk

Directions:

Take all of your ingredients and place them in an Pressure Pot Ace blender.

Process until smooth and liquified.

Nutrition: (Per serving)

Calories: 155

Protein: 7 grams

Total Fat: 2 grams

Carbohydrates: 30 grams

Blueberry Banana Protein Smoothie

Difficulty Level: 2/5

Preparation time: 5 minutes

Cooking time: 5 minutes

Servings: 1

Ingredients:

½ cup frozen and unsweetened blueberries

½ banana slices up

¾ cup plain nonfat Greek yogurt

¾ cup unsweetened vanilla almond milk

2 cups of ice cubes

Directions:

Add all of the ingredients into an Pressure Pot ace blender.

Blend until smooth.

Nutrition: (Per serving)

Calories: 230

Protein: 19.1 grams

Total Fat: 2.6 grams

Carbohydrates: 32.9 grams

Honey And Wild Blueberry Smoothie

Difficulty Level: 2/5

Preparation time: 5 minutes

Cooking time: 10 minutes

Servings: 2

Ingredients:

1 whole banana

1 cup of mango chunks

½ cup wild blueberries

½ plain, nonfat Greek yogurt

½ cup milk (for blending)

1 tablespoon raw honey

½ cup of kale

Directions:

Add all of the above ingredients into an Pressure Pot Ace blender. Add extra ice cubes if needed.

Process until smooth.

Nutrition: (Per serving)

Calories: 223

Protein: 9.4 grams

Total Fat: 1.4 grams

Carbohydrates: 46.8 grams

Oats Berry Smoothie

Difficulty Level: 2/5

Preparation time: 5 minutes

Cooking time: 5 Minutes

Servings: 2

Ingredients:

1 cup of frozen berries

1 cup Greek yogurt

¼ cup of milk

¼ cup of oats

2 teaspoon honey

Directions:

Place all ingredients in an Pressure Pot Ace blender and blend until smooth.

Nutrition: (Per serving)

Calories: 295

Protein: 18 grams

Total Fat: 5 grams

Carbohydrates: 44 grams

Kale-Pineapple Smoothie
Difficulty Level: 2/5

Preparation time: 5 minutes

Cooking time: 5 Minutes

Servings: 2

Ingredients:

1 Persian cucumber

fresh mint

1 cup of coconut milk

1 tablespoon honey

1 ½ cups of pineapple pieces

¼ pound baby kale

Directions:

Cut the ends off of the cucumbers and then cut the whole cucumber into small cubes. Strip the mint leaves from the stems.

Add all of the ingredients to your Pressure Pot Ace blender and blend until smooth.

Nutrition: (Per serving)

Calories: 140

Protein: 4 grams

Total Fat: 2.5 grams

Carbohydrates: 30 grams

Moroccan Avocado Smoothie

Difficulty Level: 2/5

Preparation time: 5 minutes

Cooking time: 0 Minutes

Servings: 4

Ingredients:

1 ripe avocado, peeled and pitted

1 overripe banana

1 cup almond milk, unsweetened

1 cup of ice

Directions:

Place the avocado, banana, milk, and ice into your Pressure Pot Ace blender.

Blend until smooth with no pieces of avocado remaining.

Nutrition: (Per serving)

Calories: 100

Protein: 1 gram

Total Fat: 6 grams

Carbohydrates: 11 grams

Mediterranean Smoothie

Difficulty Level: 2/5

Preparation time: 5 minutes

Cooking time: 5 Minutes

Servings: 2

Ingredients:

2 cups of baby spinach

1 teaspoon fresh ginger root

1 frozen banana, pre-sliced

1 small mango

½ cup beet juice

½ cup of skim milk

4-6 ice cubes

Directions:

Take all ingredients and place them in your Pressure Pot Ace blender.

Energy Value Per Serving:

Calories: 168

Protein: 4 grams

Total Fat: 1 gram

Carbohydrates: 39 grams

Anti-Inflammatory Blueberry Smoothie

Difficulty Level: 2/5

Preparation time: 5 minutes

Cooking time: 5 Minutes

Servings: 1

Ingredients:

1 cup of almond milk

1 frozen banana

1 cup frozen blueberries

2 handfuls of spinach

1 tablespoon almond butter

¼ teaspoon cinnamon

¼ teaspoon cayenne

1 teaspoon maca powder

Directions:

Combine all of these ingredients into your Pressure Pot Ace blender and blend until smooth.

Nutrition: (Per serving)

Calories: 340

Protein: 9 grams

Total Fat: 13 grams

Carbohydrates: 55 grams

Pina Colada Smoothie

Preparation Time: 10 minutes

Cooking time: 0 minutes

Servings: 4

Ingredients:

4 bananas

2 cups pineapple, peeled and sliced

2 cups mangoes, cored and diced

1 cup ice

4 tablespoons flaxseed

1¼ cups coconut milk

Directions:

Put all the ingredients in a blender and blend until smooth.

Pour into 4 glasses and immediately serve.

Nutrition:

Calories 417

Total Fat 22.1 g

Saturated Fat 17.4 g

Cholesterol 0 mg

Total Carbs 56.6 g

Dietary Fiber 9.2 g

Sugar 36.6 g

Protein 5.5 g

Kiwi Smoothie

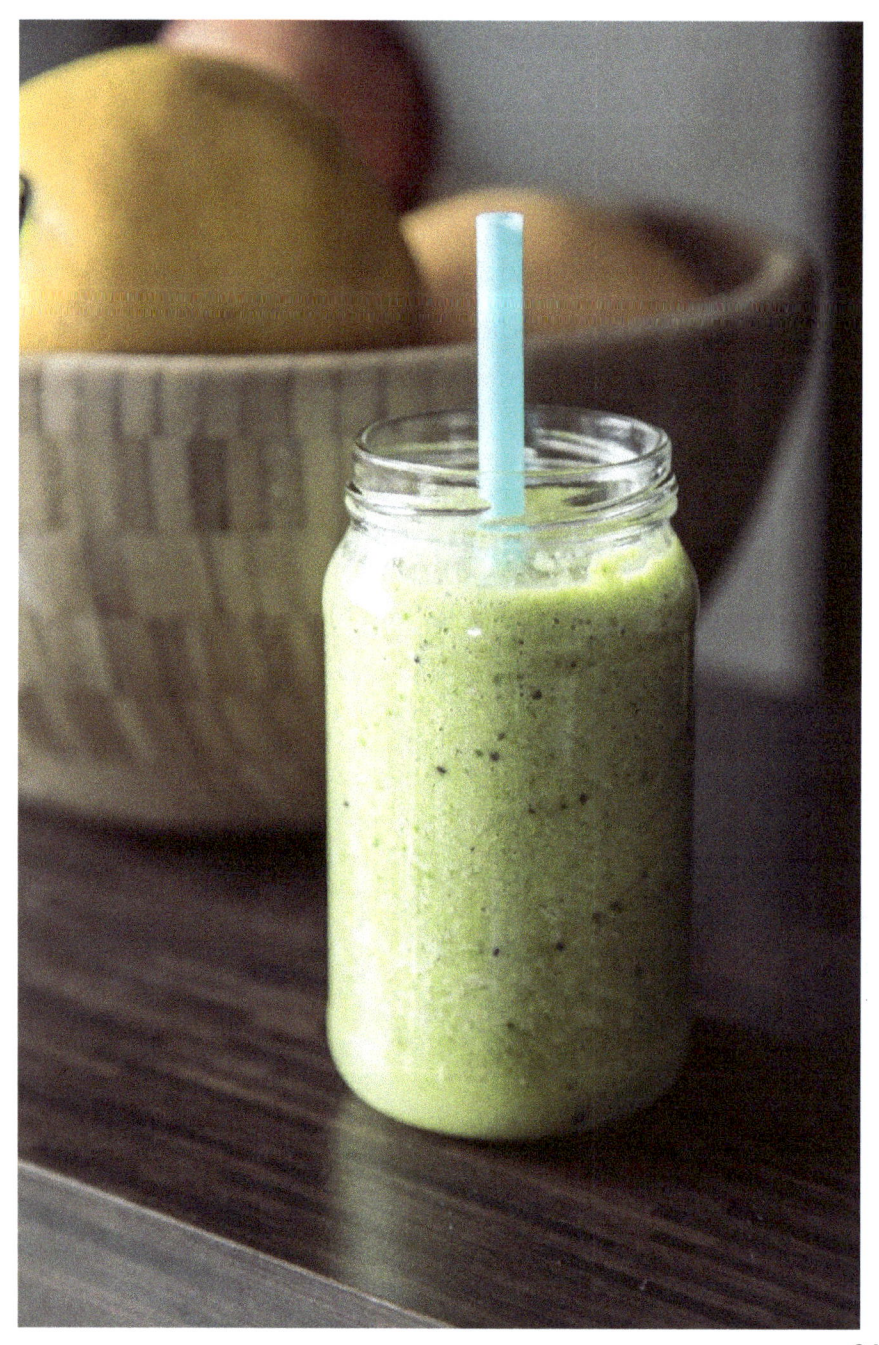

Preparation Time: *10 minutes*

Cooking time: 0 minutes

Servings: *2*

Ingredients:

1 cup basil leaves

2 bananas

1 cup fresh pineapple

10 kiwis

Directions:

Put all the ingredients in a blender and blend until smooth.

Pour into 2 glasses and immediately serve.

Nutrition:

Calories 378

Total Fat 2.5 g

Saturated Fat 0.3 g

Cholesterol 0 mg

Total Carbs 93.5 g

Dietary Fiber 15.6 g

Sugar 56.7 g

Protein 6.1 g

Whole Baked with Lemon and Herbs

Difficulty Level: 2/5

Preparation time: 10 minutes

Cooking time: 20 minutes

Servings: 4

Ingredients:

1 tablespoon olive oil, divided

2 (8-ounce) whole trout, cleaned

Sea salt

Freshly ground black pepper

1 lemon, thinly sliced into about 6 pieces

1 tablespoon finely chopped fresh dill

1 tablespoon chopped fresh parsley

½ cup low-sodium fish stock or chicken stock

Directions:

Preheat the oven to 400°F.

Lightly grease a 9-by-13-inch baking dish with 1 teaspoon of olive oil.

Rinse the trout, pat dry with paper towels, and coat with the remaining 2 teaspoons of olive oil. Season with salt and pepper.

Stuff the interior of the trout with the lemon slices, dill, and parsley and place into the prepared baking dish. Bake the fish for 10 minutes, then add the fish stock to the dish.

Continue to bake until the fish flakes easily with a fork, about 10 minutes. Serve.

Nutrition:

Calories: 194

Total fat: 10g

Saturated fat: 2g

Carbohydrates: 1g
Sugar: 0g
Fiber: 0g
Protein: 25g

Skillet Cod with Fresh Tomato Salsa

Difficulty Level: 2/5

Preparation time: 20 minutes

Cooking time: 8 minutes

Servings: 4

Ingredients:

3 tomatoes, finely chopped

1 green bell pepper, finely chopped

¼ red onion, finely chopped

¼ cup pitted, chopped green olives

2 tablespoons white wine vinegar

1 tablespoon chopped fresh basil

½ teaspoon minced garlic

4 (4-ounce) cod fillets

Sea salt

Freshly ground black pepper

1 tablespoon olive oil

Directions:

In a small bowl, stir together the tomatoes, bell pepper, onion, olives, vinegar, basil, and garlic until well mixed. Set aside.

Season the fish with salt and pepper.

In a large skillet, heat the olive oil over medium-high heat. Pan-fry the fish, turning once, until it is just cooked through, about 4 minutes per side.

Transfer to serving plates and top with a generous scoop of tomato salsa.

Nutrition:

Calories: 181

Total fat: 7g
Saturated fat: 1g;
Carbohydrates: 9g
Sugar: 4g
Fiber: 3g
Protein: 22g

Broiled Flounder with Nectarine and White Bean Salsa

Difficulty Level: 2/5

Preparation time: 20 minutes

Cooking time: 8 minutes

Servings: 4

Ingredients:

2 nectarines, pitted and chopped

1 (15-ounce) can low-sodium cannellini beans, rinsed and drained

1 red bell pepper, chopped

1 scallion, both white and green parts, chopped

2 tablespoons chopped fresh cilantro

2 tablespoons freshly squeezed lime juice

4 (4-ounce) flounder fillets

1 teaspoon smoked paprika

Sea salt

Freshly ground black pepper

Directions:

Preheat the oven to broil.

In a medium bowl, combine the nectarines, beans, bell pepper, scallion, cilantro, and lime juice.

Season the fish with paprika, salt, and pepper.

Place the fish on a baking sheet and broil, turning once, until just cooked through, about 8 minutes total. Serve the fish topped with the salsa.

Nutrition:

Calories: 259

Total fat: 8g

Saturated fat: 1g

Carbohydrates: 23g

Sugar: 8g

Fiber: 7g

Protein: 26g

Trout with Ruby Red Grapefruit Relish

Difficulty Level: 2/5

Preparation time: 15 minutes

Cooking time: 15 minutes

Servings: 4

Ingredients:

1 ruby red grapefruit, peeled, sectioned, and chopped

1 large navel orange, peeled, sectioned, and chopped

¼ English cucumber, chopped

2 tablespoons chopped red onion

1 tablespoon minced or grated lime zest

1 teaspoon minced fresh or canned peperoncino

1 teaspoon chopped fresh thyme

4 (4-ounce) trout fillets

Sea salt

Freshly ground black pepper

1 tablespoon olive oil

Directions:

Preheat the oven to 400°F.

In a medium bowl, stir together the grapefruit, orange, cucumber, onion, lime zest, peperoncino, and thyme. Cover the relish with plastic wrap and set aside in the refrigerator.

Season the trout lightly with salt and pepper and place on a baking sheet.

Brush the fish with olive oil and roast in the oven until it flakes easily with a fork, about 15 minutes. Serve topped with the chilled relish.

Nutrition:

Calories: 178

Total fat: 6g
Saturated fat: 1g
Carbohydrates: 10g
Sugar: 7g
Fiber: 2g
Protein: 25g

Classic Pork Tenderloin Marsala

Difficulty Level: 2/5

Preparation time: 10 minutes

Cooking time: 20 minutes

Servings: 4

Ingredients:

4 (3-ounce) boneless pork loin chops, trimmed

Sea salt

Freshly ground black pepper

¼ cup whole-wheat flour

1 tablespoon olive oil

2 cups sliced button mushrooms

½ sweet onion, chopped

1 teaspoon minced garlic

½ cup Marsala wine

½ cup low-sodium chicken stock

1 tablespoon cornstarch

1 tablespoon chopped fresh parsley

Directions:

Lightly season the pork chops with salt and pepper.

Pour the flour onto a plate and dredge the pork chops to coat both sides, shaking off the excess.

In a large skillet, heat the olive oil over medium-high heat and pan-fry the pork chops until cooked through and browned, turning once, about 10 minutes total. Transfer the chops to a plate and set aside.

In the skillet, combine the mushrooms, onion, and garlic and sauté until the vegetables are softened, about 5 minutes.

Stir in the wine, scraping up any bits from the skillet, and bring the liquid to a simmer.

In a small bowl, stir together the stock and cornstarch until smooth. Add the stock mixture to the skillet and bring to a boil; cook, stirring, until slightly thickened, about 4 minutes. Serve the chops with the sauce, garnished with parsley.

Nutrition:

Calories: 200

Total fat: 6g

Saturated fat: 1g

Carbohydrates: 11g

Sugar: 1g

Fiber: 1g

Protein: 20g

Chili-Spiced Lamb Chops

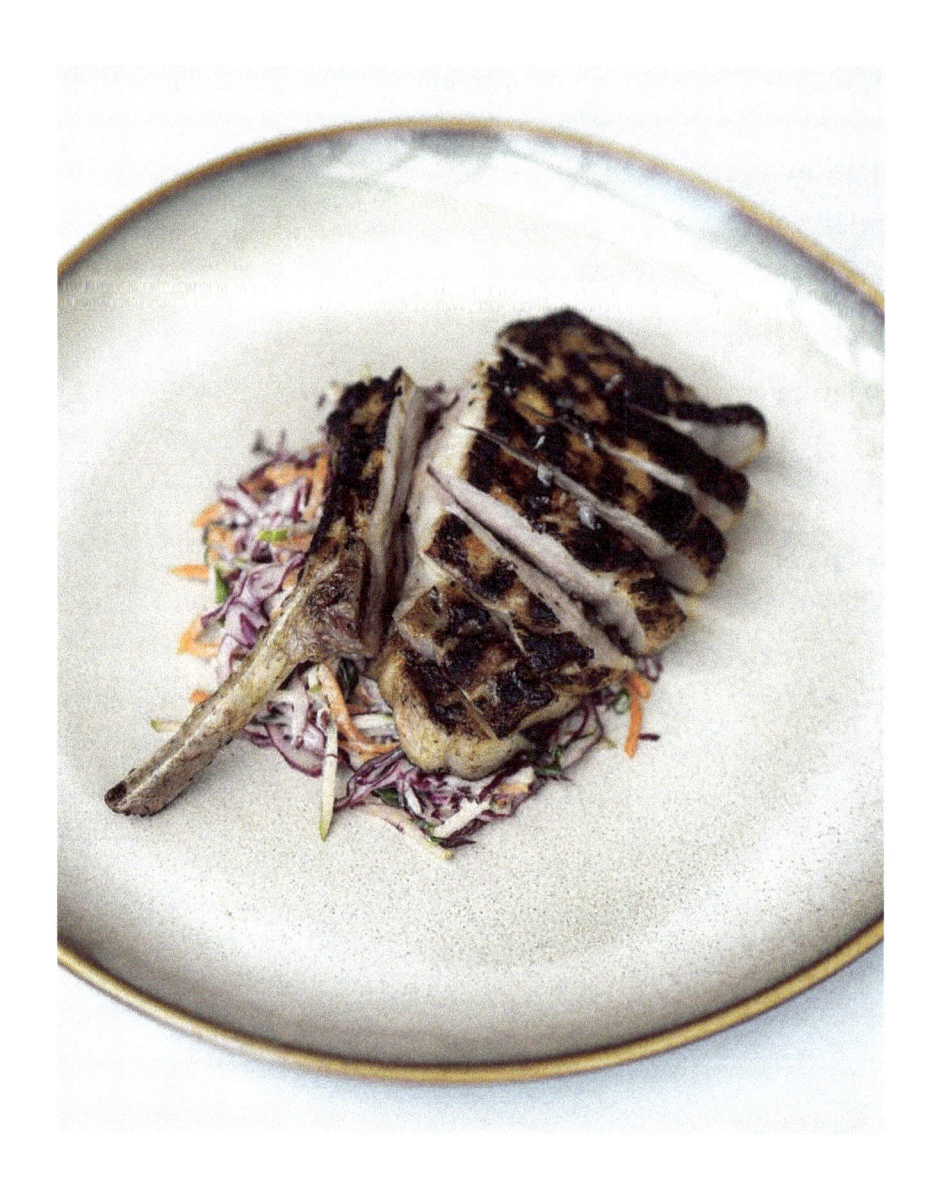

Difficulty Level: 2/5

Preparation time: 2 minutes

Cooking time: 10 minutes

Servings: 4

Ingredients:

4 (4-ounce) loin lamb chops with bones, trimmed

Sea salt

Freshly ground black pepper

1 tablespoon olive oil

2 tablespoons Sriracha sauce

1 tablespoon chopped fresh cilantro

Directions:

Preheat the oven to 450°F.

Lightly season the lamb chops with salt and pepper.

In a large ovenproof skillet, heat the olive oil over medium-high heat. Brown the chops on both sides, about 2 minutes per side, and spread the chops with sriracha.

Place the skillet in the oven and roast until the desired doneness, 4 to 5 minutes for medium. Serve topped with cilantro.

Nutrition:

Calories: 223

Total fat: 14g

Saturated fat: 4g

Carbohydrates: 1g

Sugar: 1g

Fiber: 0g

Protein: 23g

Greek Herbed Beef Meatballs

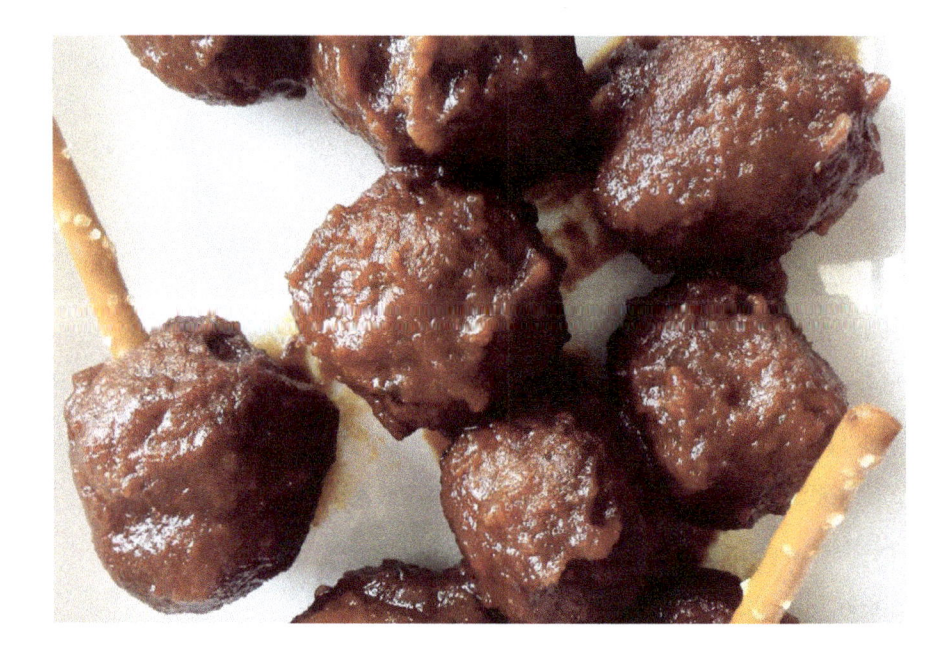

Difficulty Level: 3/5

Preparation time: 10 minutes

Cooking time: 20 minutes

Servings: 4

Ingredients:

1 pound extra-lean ground beef

½ cup panko breadcrumbs

¼ cup grated Parmesan cheese

¼ cup low-fat milk

2 large eggs

1 tablespoon chopped fresh parsley

1 teaspoon chopped fresh oregano

1 teaspoon minced garlic

¼ teaspoon freshly ground black pepper

Sea salt

Directions:

Preheat the oven to 400°F.

In a large bowl, combine the ground beef, breadcrumbs, Parmesan cheese, milk, eggs, parsley, oregano, garlic, and pepper. Season lightly with salt.

Roll the beef mixture into 1-inch meatballs and arrange on a baking sheet.

Bake the meatballs until they are cooked through and browned, turning them several times, about 20 minutes. Serve with a sauce such as Marinara Sauce or stuffed into a pita.

Nutrition:

Calories: 243

Total fat: 8g

Saturated fat: 3g

Carbohydrates: 13g

Sugar: 1g

Fiber: 2g

Protein: 24g

Sautéed Dark Leafy Greens

Difficulty Level: 2/5

Preparation time: 10 minutes

Cooking time: 10 minutes

Servings: 4

Ingredients:

2 tablespoons olive oil

8 cups stemmed and coarsely chopped spinach, kale, collard greens, or Swiss chard

Juice of ½ lemon

Sea salt

Freshly ground black pepper

Directions:

In a large skillet, heat the olive oil over medium-high heat. Add the greens and toss with tongs until wilted and tender, 8 to 10 minutes.

Remove the skillet from the heat and squeeze in the lemon juice, tossing to coat evenly. Season with salt and pepper and serve.

Nutrition:

Calories: 129

Total fat: 7g

Saturated fat: 1g

Carbohydrates: 14g

Sugar: 0g

Fiber: 2g

Protein: 4g

Lightning Source UK Ltd.
Milton Keynes UK
UKHW020734301222
414619UK00001B/11